PLANT BASED DIET COOKBOOK FOR WOMAN

50 Amazing and Mouth-watering recipes to prevent disease. Jumpstart your journey and lose weight fast with amazing dishes easy to cook and with clear instructions.

Ursa Males

TABLE OF CONTENTS

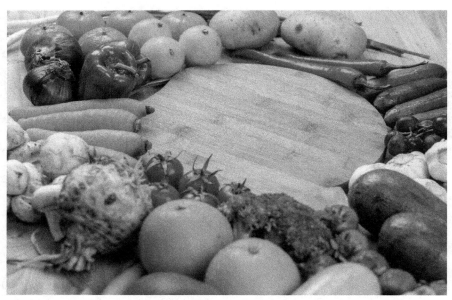

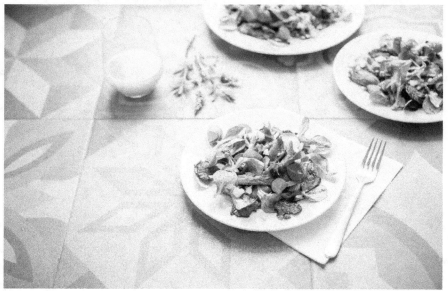

BREAKFAST

1. Skinny Peanut Butter Protein Smoothie Bowl

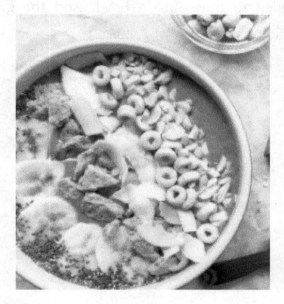

Preparation Time: 3 minutes

Cooking time: 0 minutes

Servings: 1

Ingredients:

- Granola of your preference
- 3/4 cup almond milk, unsweetened
- 1 tablespoon protein powder
- 1 tablespoon peanut butter

- 6 ice cubes
- 1/2 cup blueberries, frozen

Directions:

1. Except for the granola, add every ingredient in order into a blender and puree until smooth. Pour the blended mixture into a bowl. Add the granola as a topping.

Nutrition: Calories: 283 Carbs: 21g Protein: 22g Fat: 13g

2. **Mocha Smoothie**

Preparation Time: 5 minutes

Cooking time: 0 minutes

Servings: 2

Ingredients:

- 2 teaspoon instant espresso powder
- 2 bananas, frozen
- 1 tablespoon cocoa powder
- 1 1/2 cup soy milk

Directions:

1. Add every ingredient on the list into a blender and puree until you get a smooth mixture. Enjoy!

Nutrition: Calories: 114 Carbs: 29g Protein: 2g Fat: 1g

3. Chocolate Peanut Butter Protein Shake

Preparation Time: 5 minutes

Cooking time: 0 minutes

Servings: 1

Ingredients:

- 2 tablespoon hemp hearts
- 1 cup chocolate almond milk
- 1/4 cup peanut butter
- 2 bananas, frozen and finely minced

Directions:

1. Get a blender and throw all the Ingredients: listed above in it. Blend well until smooth.

Nutrition: Calories: 396 Carbs: 68g Protein: 14g Fat: 11g

4. <u>Breakfast Burritos</u>

Preparation Time: 10 minutes

Cooking time: 20 minutes

Servings: 1

Ingredients:

- 4 tortillas, large or burrito size
- 1 cup sliced potatoes
- 1/2 cup salsa of choice
- 1 cup nopales, minced
- Cilantro leaves, roughly diced
- 1 cup black beans, rinse and drain them
- 1 cubed avocado
- 12 oz tofu, extra firm
- Pepper, freshly ground
- Garlic
- Sea salt
- 1 teaspoon ground cumin

Directions:

1. You'll need two saucepans. Set to medium-high heat and add equal amounts of coconut oil to both pans (1 tablespoon) to let them heat.
2. To one pan, add slices of potatoes. Into the other, put the minced nopales. Sauté both.

3. The potatoes should turn a golden color, while the nopales become dry, tender, and turn a brownish color.

4. Shift your nopales to a side of the pan and add tofu. Break the tofu down using a potato masher and keep cooking. You want the tofu to turn brown too.

5. You can add the sautéed potatoes to the pan of nopales now. Also, add black beans, pepper, cumin, salt, and garlic to the pan. Stir and let the mixture cook for 5 minutes.

6. Warm your salsa of choice and tortillas. Cover the mixture in your pan, alongside your salsa and avocado with the tortillas.

Nutrition: Calories: 411 Carbs: 51g Protein: 20g Fat: 14g

5. <u>Grapes and Green Tea Smoothie</u>

Preparation time: 5 minutes

Cooking time: 0 minutes

Servings: 2

Ingredients:

- ½ cup green tea
- ½ cup of green grapes
- 1 banana, peeled
- 1-inch piece of ginger
- ½ cup of ice cubes
- 2 cups baby spinach
- ½ of a medium apple, peeled, diced

Directions:

1. Place all the fixings into the jar of a high-speed food processor or blender in the order stated in the ingredients list and then cover it with the lid.
2. Pulse for 1 minute until smooth, and then serve.

Nutrition: Calories: 150 Fat: 2.5 g Protein: 1 g Carbs: 36.5 g

6. <u>Mango and Kale Smoothie</u>

Preparation time: 5 minutes

Cooking time: 0 minutes

Servings: 2

Ingredients:

- 2 cups oats milk, unsweetened
- 2 bananas, peeled
- ½ cup kale leaves
- 2 teaspoons coconut sugar
- 1 cup mango pieces
- 1 teaspoon vanilla extract, unsweetened

Directions:

1. Place all the fixings into the jar of a high-speed food processor or blender in the order stated in the ingredients list and then cover it with the lid.
2. Pulse for 1 minute until smooth, and then serve.

Nutrition: Calories: 281 Fat: 3 g Protein: 6 g Carbs: 63 g

7. <u>Pomegranate Smoothie</u>

Preparation time: 5 minutes

Cooking time: 0 minutes

Servings: 2

Ingredients:

- 2 cups almond milk, unsweetened
- 2 medium apples, cored, sliced
- 2 bananas, peeled
- 2 cups frozen raspberries
- 1 cup pomegranate seeds
- 4 teaspoons agave syrup

Directions:

1. Place all the fixings into the jar of a high-speed food processor or blender in the order stated in the ingredients list and then cover it with the lid.
2. Pulse for 1 minute until smooth, and then serve.

Nutrition: Calories: 141.5 Fat: 1.1 g Protein: 4.1 g Carbs: 30.8 g

8. **Coconut Water Smoothie**

Preparation time: 5 minutes

Cooking time: 0 minutes

Servings: 2

Ingredients:

- 2 cups of coconut water
- 1 large apple, peeled, cored, diced
- 1 cup of frozen mango pieces
- 2 teaspoons peanut butter
- 4 teaspoons coconut flakes

Directions:

1. Place all the fixings into the jar of a high-speed food processor or blender in the order stated in the ingredients list and then cover it with the lid.
2. Pulse for 1 minute until smooth, and then serve.

Nutrition: Calories: 113.4 Fat: 0.3 g Protein: 0.6 g Carbs: 29 g

LUNCH

9. Harvest Bowl

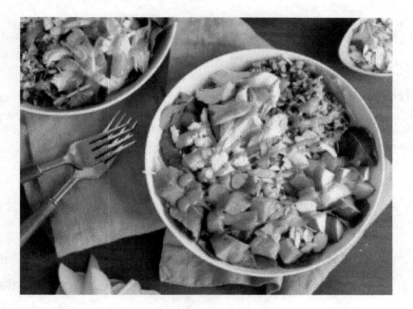

Preparation time: 15 minutes

Cooking time: 35 minutes

Servings: 4

Ingredients:

- 1 tablespoon olive oil
- 2 small sweet potatoes, chopped (about 2 cups)
- ½ teaspoon cinnamon
- ¼ teaspoon salt
- 2 cups wild rice, cooked

- 1 (14-ounce) can lentils, drained and rinsed
- 1 (14-ounce) can chickpeas, drained and rinsed
- 4 cups kale, thinly sliced and gently massaged
- 1 cup grated or shredded carrots
- ¼ cup hemp hearts
- ¼ cup raw sauerkraut (optional)
- Tahini Apple Cider Vinaigrette

Directions:

1. Warm oven to 400°F and lines a baking sheet with parchment paper. In a small bowl, mix the oil, potatoes, cinnamon, and salt.
2. Place the potatoes on the baking sheet and bake for 35 minutes or until the potatoes are nice and soft.
3. In each of 4 food storage containers, put ½ cup of rice, ¼ cup of lentils, ¼ cup of chickpeas, ¼ of the sweet potatoes, 1 cup of kale, and ¼ cup of carrots.
4. Garnish it with 1 tablespoon of hemp hearts and 1 tablespoon of sauerkraut (if using).
5. Finally, top it with 3 tablespoons of tahini vinaigrette. Cover the remaining containers with airtight lids and store them in the refrigerator.

Nutrition: Calories: 563Fat: 19gCarbohydrate: 75gProtein: 24g

10. Cauliflower Fried Rice

Preparation time: 15 minutes

Cooking time: 15 minutes

Servings: 6

Ingredients:

- 1 head cauliflower
- 1 tablespoon sesame oil
- 1 white onion, finely chopped
- 1 large carrot, finely chopped
- 4 garlic cloves, minced
- 2 cups frozen edamame or peas
- 3 scallions, sliced
- 3 tablespoons Bragg Liquid Aminos or tamari
- Salt
- Freshly ground black pepper

Directions:

1. Cut the cauliflower into florets and transfer them to a food processor. Process the cauliflower using the chopping blade and pulsing until the cauliflower is the consistency of rice. Set aside.

2. Warm a large skillet or wok over medium-high heat. Drizzle in the sesame oil and then add the onion and carrot, cooking until the carrots begin to soften about 5

minutes. Stir in the garlic and cook within another minute.

3. Add the cauliflower and edamame or peas. Heat until the cauliflower softens and the edamame or peas cook for about 5 minutes. Then add the scallions and liquid aminos or tamari. Mix well. Add in black pepper if desired.

Nutrition: Calories: 117Fat: 3gCarbohydrate: 19gProtein: 7g

11.   **<u>Curried Quinoa Salad</u>**

Preparation time: 15 minutes

Cooking time: 15 minutes

Servings: 6

Ingredients:

- 1 tablespoon olive oil
- 1 garlic clove, minced
- 1 teaspoon-sized piece of ginger, minced
- 2 teaspoons curry powder
- 1 cup quinoa, rinsed under cold water using a fine-mesh strainer
- 1½ cups vegetable broth
- 1 (14-ounce) can chickpeas, drained and rinsed
- 2 celery stalks, finely chopped
- 1 cup carrots, shredded
- ¾ cup raisins
- 1 cup cilantro, chopped
- 3 tablespoons olive oil
- 3 tablespoons apple cider vinegar
- ½ teaspoon salt
- Freshly ground black pepper

Directions:

1. Warm-up oil over medium heat in a small saucepan. Add the garlic and ginger and cook for 1 minute. Add the curry powder and stir it.

2. Next, add the quinoa and toast it for about 5 minutes, stirring regularly. Then pour in the broth, turn the heat to high, and boil.

3. Adjust your heat to simmer, cover the saucepan, and cook for about 15 minutes or until the quinoa is light and fluffy.

4. Meanwhile, in a medium bowl, combine the chickpeas, celery, carrots, raisins, and cilantro. Once the quinoa is cooked, add it to the bowl as well. Then dress it with olive oil, vinegar, salt, and as much pepper as you'd like. Mix until well combined.

Nutrition: Calories: 327Fat: 12gCarbohydrate: 50gProtein: 8g

12.   Lettuce Wraps with Smoked Tofu

Preparation time: 15 minutes

Cooking time: 25 minutes

Servings: 4

Ingredients:

- 1 (13-ounce) package organic, extra-firm smoked tofu, drained and cubed
- 1 tablespoon coconut oil
- ½ cup yellow onion, finely chopped
- 3 celery stalks, finely chopped
- 1 red bell pepper, chopped
- Pinch salt
- 1 cup cremini mushrooms, finely chopped
- 1 garlic clove, minced
- ½ teaspoon ginger, minced
- 3 tablespoons Bragg Liquid Aminos, coconut aminos, or tamari
- ½ teaspoon red pepper flakes
- Freshly ground black pepper
- 8 to 10 large romaine leaves, washed and patted dry

Directions:

1. Preheat the oven to 350°F. Prepare a baking sheet lined using parchment paper or a silicone liner; then place the tofu cubes in a single layer. Bake the tofu cubes for 25 minutes, flipping them after 10 to 15 minutes. Set aside.

2. Meanwhile, warm the coconut oil in a nonstick sauté pan over medium-high heat. Add the onion, celery, bell pepper, and salt and cook for about 5 minutes or until the onions are slightly translucent.

3. Add the mushrooms, garlic, and ginger and sauté for about 5 minutes more or until the mushrooms begin to release water. Adjust the heat to medium, then put the aminos or tamari and the red pepper flakes.

4. Add the baked tofu cubes to the pan and sprinkle with pepper. Sauté for a few minutes more, until the tofu is coated with sauce and the veggies are tender.

5. To serve, scoop as much of the veggie and tofu mixture into each romaine leaf as you'd like.

Nutrition: Calories: 160Fat: 8gCarbohydrate: 6gProtein: 14g

13. Brussels Sprouts & Cranberries Salad

Preparation Time: 10minutes

Cooking Time: 0 minute

Servings: 6

Ingredients:

- 3 tablespoons lemon juice
- ¼ cup olive oil
- Salt and pepper to taste
- 1 lb. Brussels sprouts, sliced thinly
- ¼ cup dried cranberries, chopped
- ½ cup pecans, toasted and chopped
- ½ cup Parmesan cheese shaved

Direction

1. Mix the lemon juice, olive oil, salt, and pepper in a bowl. Toss the Brussels sprouts, cranberries, and pecans in this mixture. Sprinkle the Parmesan cheese on top.

Nutrition: Calories 245 Fat 18.9 g Carbohydrate 15.9 g

Protein 6.4 g

14. Quinoa Avocado Salad

Preparation Time: 15 minutes

Cooking Time: 4 minutes

Servings: 4

Ingredients:

- 2 tablespoons balsamic vinegar
- ¼ cup cream
- ¼ cup buttermilk
- 5 tablespoons freshly squeezed lemon juice, divided
- 1 clove garlic, grated
- 2 tablespoons shallot, minced
- Salt and pepper to taste
- 2 tablespoons avocado oil, divided
- 1 ¼ cups quinoa, cooked
- 2 heads endive, sliced
- 2 firm pears, sliced thinly
- 2 avocados, sliced
- ¼ cup fresh dill, chopped

Direction

1. Combine the vinegar, cream, milk, 1 tablespoon lemon juice, garlic, shallot, salt, and pepper in a bowl. Pour 1 tablespoon oil into a pan over medium heat. Heat the quinoa for 4 minutes.

2. Transfer quinoa to a plate. Toss the endive and pears in a mixture of remaining oil, remaining lemon juice, salt, and pepper. Transfer to a plate.
3. Toss the avocado in the reserved dressing. Add to the plate. Top with the dill and quinoa.

Nutrition: Calories: 431 Fat: 28.5g Carbohydrates: 42.7g Protein:6.6g

15. <u>Roasted Sweet Potatoes</u>

Preparation Time: 20 minutes

Cooking Time: 20 minutes

Servings: 4

Ingredients:

- 2 potatoes, sliced into wedges
- 2 tablespoons olive oil, divided
- Salt and pepper to taste
- 1 red bell pepper, chopped
- ¼ cup fresh cilantro, chopped
- 1 garlic, minced
- 2 tablespoons almonds, toasted and sliced
- 1 tablespoon lime juice

Directions:

1. Warm your oven to 425 degrees F. Toss the sweet potatoes in oil and salt. Transfer to a baking pan. Roast for 20 minutes.

2. In a bowl, combine the red bell pepper, cilantro, garlic, and almonds. In another bowl, mix the lime juice, remaining oil, salt, and pepper.

3. Drizzle this mixture over the red bell pepper mixture. Serve sweet potatoes with the red bell pepper mixture.

Nutrition: Calories: 146 Fat: 8.6g   Carbohydrates: 16g Protein:2.3g

16. Farro and Lentil Salad

Preparation time: 10 minutes

Cooking time: 0 minutes

Servings: 4

Ingredients:

For the Salad:

- 1 cup grape tomato, halved
- ½ cup diced yellow bell pepper
- 1 cup diced cucumber,
- ½ cup diced red bell pepper
- 1 cup fresh arugula
- 1/3 cup chopped parsley
- 1 ½ cups lentils, cooked
- 3 ½ cups farro, cooked
- For the Dressing:
- ½ teaspoon minced garlic
- ½ teaspoon salt
- ¼ teaspoon ground black pepper
- 1 teaspoon Italian seasoning
- 1 teaspoon Dijon mustard
- 2 tablespoons red wine vinegar
- 2 tablespoons lemon juice
- 1/3 cup olive oil

Directions:

1. Take a large bowl, place all the ingredients for the salad except for arugula and then toss until combined.
2. Prepare the dressing and for this, take a medium bowl, add all of its ingredients in it and then stir whisk until well combined.
3. Pour the dressing over the salad, toss until well coated, then distribute salad among four bowls and top with arugula. Serve straight away.

Nutrition: Cal 379 Fat 10 g Carbohydrates 63.5 g Protein 12.5 g

17.   Greek Zoodle Bowl

Preparation time: 10 minutes

Cooking time: 0 minutes

Servings: 4

Ingredients:

- ½ cup chopped artichokes
- 14 cherry tomatoes, chopped
- 1 medium red bell peppers, cored, chopped
- 4 medium zucchinis
- 1 medium yellow bell pepper, cored, chopped
- 6 tablespoons hemp hearts
- 1 English cucumber
- 6 tablespoons chopped red onion
- 2 tablespoons chopped parsley leaves
- 2 tablespoons chopped mint
- For the Greek Dressing:
- 2 tablespoons chopped mint
- 1 teaspoon garlic powder
- ½ teaspoon salt
- ¼ teaspoon dried oregano
- 2 teaspoons Italian seasoning
- 3 tablespoons red wine vinegar
- 1 tablespoon olive oil

Directions:

1. Prepare zucchini and cucumber noodles, spiralize them using a spiralizer or vegetable peeler and then divide evenly among four bowls.
2. Top zucchini and cucumber noodles with artichokes, tomato, bell pepper, hemp hearts, onion, parsley, and mint, and then set aside until required.
3. Prepare the dressing, take a small bowl, add all the ingredients for the dressing, and whisk until combined.
4. Add the prepared dressing evenly into each bowl, then toss until the vegetables are well coated with the dressing and serve.

Nutrition: Cal 250 Fat 14 g Carbohydrates 19 g Protein 13 g

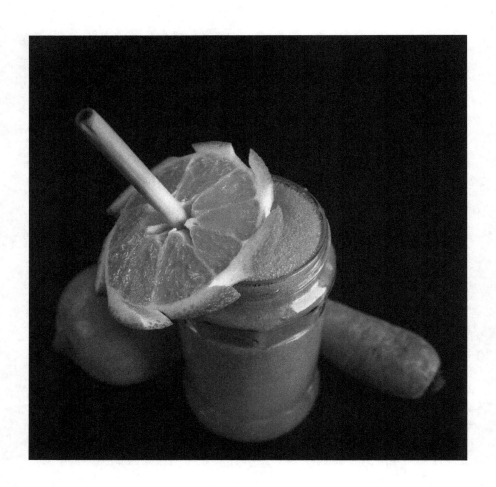

DINNER

18.   Vegetables with Wild Rice

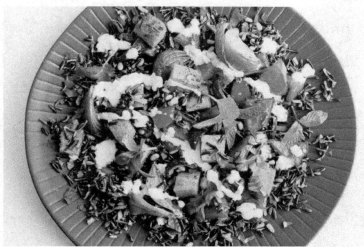

Preparation time: 15 minutes

Cooking time: 0 minutes

Servings: 4

Ingredients:

- Salt
- Basil
- Cilantro
- Juice of one lime
- 1 Chopped chili pepper
- ½ cup Vegetable broth
- 1 cup Bean sprouts

- 2 cups Chopped carrots
- 1 cup Beans – green - diced
- 1 cup Broccoli, cleaved
- 1 cup Pak Choi
- 1 cup Wild rice

Directions:

1. Place all the chopped vegetables into a pan and add vegetable broth. Steam fries the vegetables until they are cooked through but still crunchy.
2. Using a mortar and pestle grind up the chili, basil, and cilantro until it forms a paste. Add in lime juice and mix well.
3. Place the rice onto a serving platter. Add the vegetables on top and drizzle with dressing.

Nutrition: Calories: 376 Carbs: 55g Fat: 15g Protein: 0g

19. Tangy Lentil Soup

Preparation time: 15 minutes

Cooking time: 10 minutes

Servings: 4

Ingredients:

- salt
- ¼ tsp turmeric
- 3 cloves minced garlic
- 1 1/2-inch grated ginger
- 1 chopped tomato
- 1 chopped serrano chili pepper
- 2 cups rinsed red lentils

Topping:

- ¼ cup Coconut yogurt

Directions:

1. Place the lentils in a colander and place under running water. Rinse until free from dirt and stones.
2. Pour rinsed lentils into a pot. Add enough water to cover lentils. Place the pot over medium heat and allow to boil.

3. Lower heat and simmer for 10 minutes. Put in the leftover contents then mix properly to blend. Still, cook until lentils are soft. Garnish with a spoonful of coconut yogurt.

Nutrition: Calories: 240 Carbs: 38g Fat: 3g Protein: 20g

20. <u>Mushroom Leek Soup</u>

Preparation time: 15 minutes

Cooking time: 20 minutes

Servings: 4

Ingredients:

- 1 ½ tbsp sherry vinegar
- ½ cup almond milk
- ¾ cup coconut cream
- 3 cups vegetable broth
- 1 tbsp chopped dill
- pepper
- salt
- 5 tbsp almond flour
- 7 cups cleaned, sliced mushrooms
- 3 cloves minced garlic
- 2 ¾ cups chopped leeks
- 3 tbsp vegetable oil

Directions:

1. Place a Dutch oven on medium and warm the oil. Add in the leeks together with garlic bulb then prepare till soft. Put in the mushrooms, stir and cook an additional 10 minutes.

2. Add salt, dill, pepper, and flour. Stir well, until combined. Put in soup and cause it to simmer. Lessen heat and put in rest of the ingredients. Stir well. Cook an additional 10 minutes. Serve warm with almond flour bread.

Nutrition: Calories: 117 Carbs: 19g Fat: 2g Protein: 3g

21. Fresh Veggie Pizza

Preparation time: 15 minutes

Cooking time: 14 minutes

Servings: 4

Ingredients:

Crust:

- ½ tsp Garlic bulb flavored powder
- ½ tsp Seawater salt
- 3 tbsp Coconut oil
- 1 ¼ cup Almond flour

Tahini-Bee Spread:

- Pepper, pinch
- Sea salt, pinch
- 2 cloves Garlic
- 1 tbsp Juice - Lemon
- 1 tbsp Avocado oil
- 1 tbsp Middle eastern paste
- 2 Peeled and cubed beets

Directions:

1. Start by placing your oven to 375. Place some parchment on a sheet tray. Stir together the salt, garlic powder, coconut oil, and almond flour.

2. Place this on the sheet tray and squeeze into the shape of a ball. Place another piece of parchment on top and roll out the dough into 7x7 square. Bake for 14 minutes, or until it starts to brown.

3. As the crust bakes, add the pepper, salt, garlic, lemon juice, avocado oil, tahini, and beets to a food processor. Mix until it becomes creamy.

4. To make your pizza, spread the crust with beet sauces and then top with your favorite alkaline friendly veggies. Slice into four and enjoy.

Nutrition: Calories: 368 Carbs: 46g Fat: 13g Protein: 16g

22. <u>Spicy Lentil Burgers</u>

Preparation time: 15 minutes

Cooking time: 20 minutes

Servings: 4

Ingredients:

- 1 tbsp avocado oil
- 1 tbsp coconut flour
- 2 cloves crushed garlic
- diced jalapeno
- ½ cup chopped cilantro
- ½ cup diced onion
- ½ tsp pepper
- ½ tsp sea salt
- ½ cup almond flour
- ½ cup dry lentils

Directions:

1. Cook the lentils following the directions on the package and set them to the side to cool off.
2. Mix together the garlic, jalapeno, cilantro, onion, pepper, salt, almond flour, and lentils until everything is well combined.
3. Add half of the lentil mixture to a food processor and process until it reaches a paste-like consistency.

4. Pour this back into the bowl with the rest of the lentil mixture and stir everything together. The mixture will be very moist. Stir in the coconut flour to help get rid of the moisture and to help them hold together.

5. Divide the mixture into fourths. Squeeze one-fourth of the mixture in your hands to flatten it out into a burger shape. Do this for the three remaining sections.

6. Warm up the oil in an exceedingly massive pot and put in the burgers. Prepare the burgers on 4 to 6 minutes on both sides, or until they have turned golden.

7. When you flip them, do so carefully so that they don't fall apart. Enjoy.

Nutrition: Calories: 103 Carbs: 18g Fat: 1g Protein: 6g

23. Roasted Cauliflower Wraps

Preparation time: 15 minutes

Cooking time: 30-35 minutes

Servings: 2

Ingredients:

Cauliflower:

- ¼ tsp pepper
- ¼ tsp sea salt
- ½ tsp garlic powder
- ¼ cup nutritional yeast
- ¼ cup almond flour
- 1 tbsp avocado oil
- 2 cups bite-size cauliflower florets

Sauce:

- sea salt
- 2 tbsp apple cider vinegar
- 2 cloves garlic
- habanero pepper
- 1 cup cubed mango

Assembling:

- 2 leaves collard greens
- 1 cup mixed salad greens.

Directions:

1. Start by placing your kitchen appliance to 350 degrees then put a few papers on a cooking film. For your cauliflower, toss the cauliflower in the avocado oil and make sure they are evenly coated.

2. Into a container, combine along the all the pepper, salt, garlic powder, healthy fungus, together with the almond flour.

3. Sprinkle the breading over the cauliflower and toss everything together making sure that the cauliflower is well-coated. Spread across the cooking film.

4. Cook it on about 30 up to 35 minutes, either that or till the cauliflower is soft.

5. As the cauliflower bakes, add the salt, vinegar, garlic, habanero, and mango to your blender and mix until well-combined.

6. Make sure that you use some gloves or wash your hands really well when it comes to handling the habanero.

7. To assemble, divide the mixed salad greens between the collard leaves, top with the cauliflower and drizzle on the sauce.

8. Wrap everything up like a burrito and enjoy.

Nutrition: Calories: 270 Carbs: 14g Fat: 22g Protein: 6g

24. Sliced Sweet Potato with Artichoke and Pepper Spread

Preparation time: 15 minutes

Cooking time: 45 minutes

Servings: 4

Ingredients:

- ¼ tsp pepper
- ½ tsp salt
- 6 tsp avocado oil, divided
- quartered red bell pepper
- 2 unpeeled sweet potatoes, sliced into 4 lengthwise slices
- 2 cloves garlic
- 1 can (14 oz) artichoke hearts

Directions:

1. Start by placing the oven to 350. Place some parchment on a sheet tray and set to the side.
2. Lay the bell pepper and sweet potato on the sheet tray and top them with two teaspoons of avocado oil, a pinch of pepper, and a pinch of salt. Bake them for 30 minutes. Turn it over and cook to an additional 15 minutes.

3. Add the roasted red bell pepper to a food processor along with the garlic, artichoke hearts, pepper, salt, and the remaining avocado oil.
4. Pulse until combined but still a little chunky. Adjust any seasonings that you need. Top the slices of sweet potato with the spread and enjoy.

Nutrition: Calories: 670 Carbs: 39g Fat: 39g Protein: 43g

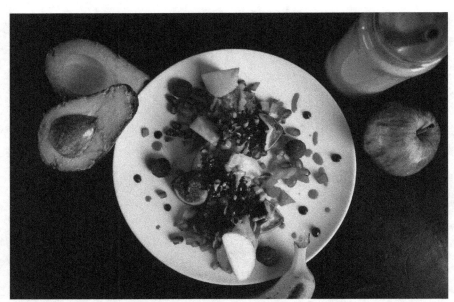

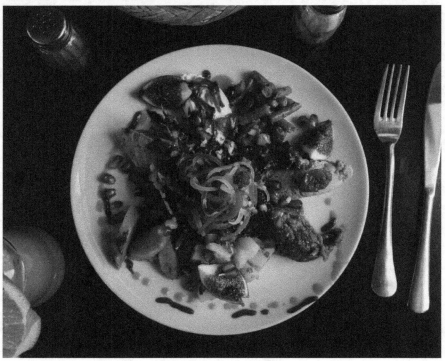

SNACKS

25. Banana Nut Bread Bars

Preparation Time: 5 Minutes

Cooking Time: 30 Minutes

Servings: 9

Ingredients:

- Nonstick cooking spray (optional)
- 2 large ripe bananas
- 2 tablespoon maple syrup
- ½ teaspoon vanilla extract
- 2 cups old-fashioned rolled oats
- ½ teaspoons salt
- ¼ cup chopped walnuts

Directions:

1. Preheat the oven to 350°F. Lightly coat a 9-by-9-inch baking pan with nonstick cooking spray (if using) or line with parchment paper for oil-free baking.
2. In a medium bowl, mash the bananas with a fork. Add the maple syrup and vanilla extract and mix well. Add the oats, salt, and walnuts, mixing well.

3. Move the batter to the baking pan and bake for 25 to 30 minutes, until the top is crispy. Cool completely before slicing into 9 bars. Transfer to an airtight storage container or a large plastic bag.

Nutrition: Calories: 73Fat: 1gCarbohydrates: 15gProtein: 2g

26. <u>Rosemary and Lemon Zest Popcorn</u>

Preparation Time: 10 Minutes

Cooking Time: 0 Minutes

Servings: 2

Ingredients:

- 1/3 cup popcorn kernels
- 2 tablespoon vegan butter, melted
- 1 tablespoon chopped rosemary
- 1 teaspoon lemon zest
- ¼ teaspoon salt

Directions:

1. Pop the kernels, and when done, transfer them into a large bowl. Drizzle butter over the popcorns, sprinkle with salt, lemon zest, and rosemary, and then toss until combined. Serve straight away.

Nutrition: Calories: 201Protein: 3gCarbohydrates: 25g

Fats: 10g

27. **<u>Strawberry Avocado Toast</u>**

Preparation Time: 5 Minutes

Cooking Time: 0 Minutes

Servings: 4

Ingredients:

- 1 avocado, peeled, pitted, and quartered
- 4 whole-wheat bread slices, toasted
- 4 ripe strawberries, cut into ¼-inch slices
- 1 tablespoon balsamic glaze or reduction

Directions:

1. Mash one-quarter of your avocado on a slice of toast. Put one-quarter of the strawberry slices over your avocado, then finish with a drizzle of balsamic glaze. Repeat with the remaining fixings, and serve.

Nutrition: Calories: 150Fats: 8gCarbohydrates: 17gProtein: 5g

28. <u>**Strawberry Watermelon Ice Pops**</u>

Preparation Time: 6 Hours & 5 Minutes

Cooking Time: 0 Minutes

Servings: 6

Ingredients:

- 4 cups diced watermelon
- 4 strawberries, tops removed
- 2 tablespoons freshly squeezed lime juice

Directions:

1. Combine the watermelon, strawberries, and lime juice in a blender. Blend within 1 to 2 minutes, or until well combined.
2. Pour evenly into 6 ice-pop molds, insert ice-pop sticks, and freeze for at least 6 hours before serving.

Nutrition: Calories: 61Fat: 0gCarbohydrates: 15gProtein: 1g

29. <u>Carrot Energy Balls</u>

Preparation Time: 10 Minutes

Cooking Time: 0 Minutes

Servings: 8

Ingredients:

- 1 large carrot, grated carrot
- 1 ½ cups old-fashioned oats
- 1 cup raisins
- 1 cup dates, pitied
- 1 cup coconut flakes
- 1/4 teaspoon ground cloves
- 1/2 teaspoon ground cinnamon

Directions:

1. Pulse all fixings in your food processor until it forms a sticky and uniform mixture. Shape the batter into equal balls. Place in your refrigerator until ready to serve. Bon appétit!

Nutrition: Calories: 495Protein: 22gCarbohydrates: 58g Fat: 21g

VEGETABLES

30. <u>Whipped Potatoes</u>

Preparation Time: 20 minutes

Cooking Time: 35 minutes

Servings: 10

Ingredients:

- 4 cups water
- 3 lb. potatoes, sliced into cubes
- 3 cloves garlic, crushed
- 6 tablespoons butter
- 2 bay leaves
- 10 sage leaves
- ½ cup Greek yogurt
- ¼ cup low-Fat milk

Direction

1. Cook potatoes in water for 30 minutes.
2. Drain.
3. Cook garlic in butter for 1 minute over medium heat.
4. Add the sage and cook for 5 more minutes.
5. Discard the garlic.
6. Use a fork to mash the potatoes.

7. Whip using an electric mixer while gradually adding the butter, yogurt, and milk.

8. Season with salt.

Nutrition: 169 Calories 22g Carbohydrates 4.2g Protein

31. <u>Jalapeno Rice Noodles</u>

Preparation Time: 10 minutes

Cooking Time: 25 minutes

Servings: 4

Ingredients

- ¼ cup soy sauce
- 1 tablespoon brown sugar
- 2 teaspoons sriracha
- 3 tablespoons lime juice
- 8 oz rice noodles
- 3 teaspoons toasted sesame oil
- 1 package extra-firm tofu, pressed
- 1 onion, sliced
- 2 cups green cabbage, shredded
- 1 small jalapeno, minced
- 1 red bell pepper, sliced
- 1 yellow bell pepper, sliced
- 3 garlic cloves, minced
- 3 scallions, sliced
- 1 cup Thai basil leaves, roughly chopped

- Lime wedges for serving

Directions:

1. Fill a suitably-sized pot with salted water and boil it on high heat.
2. Add pasta to the boiling water and cook until it is al dente, then rinse under cold water.
3. Put lime juice, soy sauce, sriracha, and brown sugar in a bowl then mix well.
4. Place a large wok over medium heat then add 1 teaspoon sesame oil.
5. Toss in tofu and stir for 5 minutes until golden-brown.
6. Transfer the golden-brown tofu to a plate and add 2 teaspoons oil to the wok.
7. Stir in scallions, garlic, peppers, cabbage, and onion.
8. Sauté for 2 minutes, then add cooked noodles and prepared sauce.
9. Cook for 2 minutes, then garnish with lime wedges and basil leaves.

10. Serve fresh.

Nutrition: Calories:45 Fat:2.5g Protein:4g Carbohydrates:9g
Fiber:4g Sugar:3g Sodium: 20mg

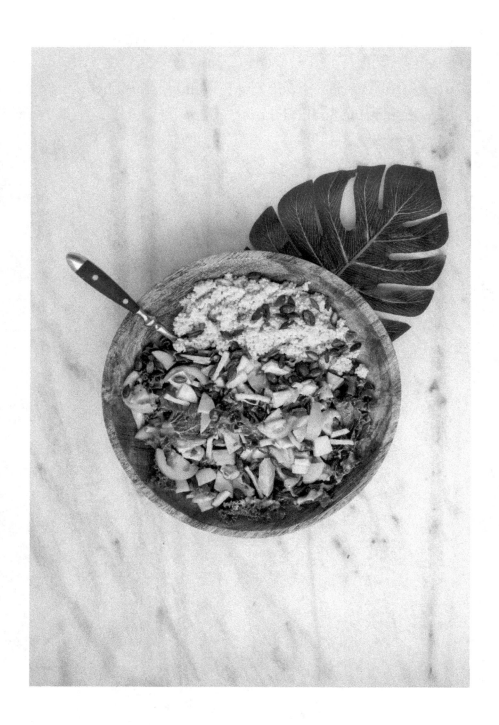

SALAD

32. <u>Sautéed Cabbage</u>

Preparation Time: 8 minutes

Cooking Time: 12 minutes

Servings: 8

Ingredients:

- ¼ cup butter
- 1 onion, sliced thinly
- 1 head cabbage, sliced into wedges
- Salt and pepper to taste
- Crumbled crispy bacon bits

Instructions:

1. Add the butter to a pan over medium high heat.
2. Cook the onion for 1 minute, stirring frequently.
3. Season with the salt and pepper.
4. Add the cabbage and cook while stirring for 12 minutes.
5. Sprinkle with the crispy bacon bits.

Nutrition: Calories 77 Fat 5.9 g Saturated fat 3.6 g

Carbohydrates 6.1 g Fiber 2.4 g Protein 1.3 g

33. Southwest Style Salad

Preparation Time: 10 minutes

Cooking Time: 0 minutes

Servings: 3

Ingredients:

- ½ cup dry black beans
- ½ cup dry chickpeas
- 1/3 cup purple onion, diced
- 1 red bell pepper, pitted, sliced
- 4 cups mixed greens, fresh or frozen, chopped
- 1 cup cherry tomatoes, halved or quartered
- 1 medium avocado, peeled, pitted, and cubed
- 1 cup sweet kernel corn, canned, drained
- ½ tsp. chili powder
- ¼ tsp. cumin
- ¼ tsp Salt
- ¼ tsp pepper
- 2 tsp. olive oil
- 1 tbsp. vinegar

Directions:

1. Prepare the black beans and chickpeas according to the method.
2. Put all of the ingredients into a large bowl.

3. Toss the mix of veggies and spices until combined thoroughly.
4. Store, or serve chilled with some olive oil and vinegar on top!

Nutrition: Calories 635Total Fat 19.9gSaturated Fat 3.6g

Cholesterol 0mgSodium 302mgTotal Carbohydrate 95.4g

Dietary Fiber 28.1gTotal Sugars 18.8gProtein 24.3gVitamin D 0mcgCalcium 160mgIron 7mgPotassium 1759mg

GRAINS

34. <u>Sweet Potato and White Bean Skillet</u>

Preparation Time: 5 minutes

Cooking Time: 20 minutes

Servings: 4

Ingredients:

- 1 bunch kale, chopped
- 2 sweet potatoes, peeled, cubed
- 12 oz. cannellini beans
- 1 peeled onion, diced
- 1/8 tsp. red pepper flakes
- 1 tsp. salt
- 1 tsp. cumin
- ½ tsp. ground black pepper
- 1 tsp. curry powder
- 1 ½ tbsps. coconut oil
- 6 oz. coconut milk, unsweetened

Directions:

1. Take a large skillet pan, place it over medium heat, add ½ tablespoon oil and when it melts, add onion and cook for 5 minutes.

2. Then stir in sweet potatoes, stir well, cook for 5 minutes, then season with all the spices, cook for 1 minute and remove the pan from heat.

3. Take another pan, add remaining oil in it, place it over medium heat and when oil melts, add kale, season with some salt and black pepper, stir well, pour in the milk and cook for 15 minutes until tender.

4. Then add beans, beans, and red pepper, stir until mixed and cook for 5 minutes until hot.

5. Serve straight away.

Nutrition: Calories: 263, Fat: 4 g, Carbs: 44 g, Protein: 13 g

35. <u>Veggie Kabobs</u>

Preparation Time: 10 minutes

Cooking Time: 10 minutes

Servings: 10

Ingredients:

- 8 oz. button mushrooms, halved
- 2 lbs. summer squash, peeled, 1-inch cubed
- 12 oz. small broccoli florets
- 2 c. grape tomatoes
- 1 tsp. salt
- ½ tsp. smoked paprika
- 1 tsp. ground cumin
- 6 tbsps. olive oil
- 1/2 tsp. ground coriander
- 1 lime, juiced

Directions:

1. Toss broccoli florets with 1 tablespoon oil, toss tomatoes and squash pieces with 2 tablespoons oil, toss mushrooms with 1 tablespoon oil and thread these vegetables onto skewers.
2. Grill mushrooms and broccoli for 7 to 10 minutes, squash and tomatoes and 8 minutes, and when done,

transfer the skewers to a plate and drizzle with lime juice and remaining oil.

3. Prepared the spice mix and for this, stir together salt, paprika, cumin, and coriander, sprinkle half of the mixture over grilled veggies, cover them with foil for 5 minutes, and then sprinkle with the remaining spice mix.

4. Serve straight away.

Nutrition: Calories: 110, Fat: 9 g, Carbs: 8 g, Protein: 3 g

LEGUMES

36. Black-Eyed Pea Salad (Ñebbe)

Preparation Time: 10 minutes

Cooking Time: 10 minutes

Servings: 4

Ingredients:

- 2 cups dried black-eyed peas, soaked overnight and drained
- 2 tablespoons basil leaves, chopped
- 2 tablespoons parsley leaves, chopped
- 1 shallot, chopped
- 1 cucumber, sliced
- 2 bell peppers, seeded and diced
- 1 Scotch bonnet chili pepper, seeded and finely chopped
- 1 cup cherry tomatoes, quartered
- Sea salt and ground black pepper, to taste
- 2 tablespoons fresh lime juice
- 1 tablespoon apple cider vinegar
- 1/4 cup extra-virgin olive oil
- 1 avocado, peeled, pitted and sliced

Directions

1. Cover the black-eyed peas with water by 2 inches and bring to a gentle boil. Let it boil for about 15 minutes.
2. Then, turn the heat to a simmer for about 45 minutes. Let it cool completely.
3. Place the black-eyed peas in a salad bowl. Add in the basil, parsley, shallot, cucumber, bell peppers, cherry tomatoes, salt and black pepper.
4. In a mixing bowl, whisk the lime juice, vinegar and olive oil.
5. Dress the salad, garnish with fresh avocado and serve immediately. Bon appétit!

Nutrition: Calories: 471; Fat: 17.5g; Carbs: 61.5g; Protein: 20.6g

BREAD & PIZZA

37. Almond Bread

Preparation Time: 10 Minutes

Cooking Time: 30 Minutes

Servings: 20

Ingredients:

- Eggs – 6, separated
- Cream of tartar – 1/4 teaspoon.
- Baking powder – 3 teaspoons.
- Butter – 4 tablespoons, melted
- Almond flour – 1 1/2 cups
- Salt – 1/4 teaspoon.

Directions:

1. Preheat the oven to 375 F. Grease 8*4-inch loaf pan with butter and set aside. Add egg whites and cream of tartar in a large bowl and beat until soft peaks form.
2. Add almond flour, baking powder, egg yolks, butter, and salt in a food processor and process until combined.
3. Add 1/3 of egg white mixture into the almond flour mixture and process until combined. Now add

remaining egg white mixture and process gently to combine.

4. Pour batter into the prepared loaf pan and bake for 30 minutes. Slice and serve.

Nutrition: Calories 52, Carbs 1g, Fat 4g, Protein 2g

SOUP AND STEW

38. Beet and Kale Salad

Preparation Time: 5 minutes

Cooking Time: 5 minutes

Servings: 1

Ingredients:

- 8 ounces of beet and kale blend
- 1 tablespoon of olive oil
- 1 cucumber
    - ounce of chickpeas
- Salt
- 2 tablespoons of red wine vinegar
- Pepper - ¼ cup of walnuts
- 2 ounces of dried cranberries
- Cashew cheese

Directions:

1. Cut the veggies and combine everything in a big salad bowl.
2. Serve the fresh salad and enjoy a hearty meal.

Nutrition: kcal: 490 Carbohydrates: 31 g Protein: 19 g Fat: 21 g

39. Kale and Cauliflower Salad

Preparation Time: 10 minutes

Cooking Time: 15 minutes

Servings: 1 portion

Ingredients:

- 6 ounces of Lacinato kale
- 8 ounces of cauliflower florets
- 1 lemon
- 1 tablespoon of Italian spice
- 2 radishes
- ounce of butter beans
- Olive oil
- ¼ cup of walnuts
- ¼ cup of vegan Caesar dressing
- Pepper
- Salt

Directions:

1. Preheat the oven to 400°F. Put the cauliflower florets on a baking sheet, toss them with olive oil and spices, and add salt. Roast the cauliflower until it is brown. It will be done within 15-20 minutes.

2. De-stem the kale and slice the leaves. Slice the radishes. Both kale and radish should be sliced thinly. Cut the lemon in half.

3. Put the kale in a large bowl and add the lemon juice and salt along with the pepper. Massage the kale so that it is properly covered with seasoning. The leaves will soon turn dark green. Mix the radishes.

4. Rinse the butter beans and pat them dry with a towel. On medium-high heat, put a large skillet, add some olive oil, and sauté the butter beans in a layer. Sprinkle some salt on top and shake the pan. The butter beans will be brown in places within 7 minutes.

5. Take two large plates and divide both the kale and beans equally. Put the walnuts and roasted cauliflower on top. Add the Caesar dressing on top and enjoy the amazing salad.

Nutrition: kcal: 378 Carbohydrates: 11 g Protein: 18 g Fat: 27 g

40. <u>Maple Dijon Dressing</u>

Preparation Time: 5 minutes

Cooking Time: 0 minutes

Servings: 1

Ingredients:

- ¼ cup apple cider vinegar
- 2 teaspoons Dijon mustard
- 2 tablespoons maple syrup
- 2 tablespoons low-sodium vegetable broth
- ¼ teaspoon black pepper
- Salt, to taste (optional)

Directions:

1. Mix the apple cider vinegar, Dijon mustard, maple syrup, vegetable broth, and black pepper in a resealable container until well incorporated. Season with salt to taste, if desired.
2. The dressing can be refrigerated for up to 5 days.

Nutrition: calories: 82fat: 0.3gcarbs: 19.3gprotein: 0.6g fiber: 0.7g

41. <u>Avocado-Chickpea Dip</u>

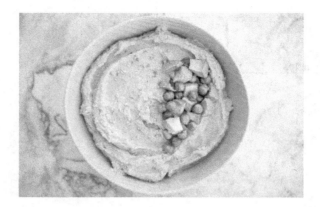

Preparation Time: 15 minutes

Cooking Time: 0 minutes

Servings: 2

Ingredients:

- 1 (15-ounce / 425-g) can cooked chickpeas, drained and rinsed
- 2 large, ripe avocados, chopped
- ¼ cup red onion, finely chopped
- 1 tablespoon Dijon mustard
- 1 to 2 tablespoons lemon juice
- 2 teaspoons chopped fresh oregano
- 1/2 teaspoon garlic clove, finely chopped

Directions:

1. In a medium bowl, mash the cooked chickpeas with a potato masher or the back of a fork, or until the

chickpeas pop open (a food processor works best for this).

2. Stir in the remaining ingredients and continue to mash until completely smooth.

3. Place in the refrigerator to chill until ready to serve.

Nutrition: calories: 101fat: 1.9gcarbs: 16.2g protein: 4.7gfiber: 4.6g

APPETIZER

42. <u>Kale Chips</u>

Preparation time: 5 minutes

Cooking time: 25 minutes

Servings: 2

Ingredients:

- 1 large bunch kale
- 1 tablespoon extra-virgin olive oil
- ½ teaspoon chipotle powder
- ½ teaspoon smoked paprika
- ¼ teaspoon salt

Directions:

1. Preheat the oven to 275°F. Prepare a large baking sheet lined using parchment paper. In a large bowl, stem the kale and tear it into bite-size pieces. Add the olive oil, chipotle powder, smoked paprika, and salt.
2. Toss the kale with tongs or your hands, coating each piece well. Spread the kale over the parchment paper in a single layer.

3. Bake within 25 minutes, turning halfway through, until crisp. Cool for 10 to 15 minutes before dividing and storing in 2 airtight containers.

Nutrition: Calories: 100 Carbs: 9g Fat: 7g Protein: 4g

43. <u>Tempeh-Pimiento Cheese Ball</u>

Preparation time: 5 minutes

Cooking time: 30 minutes

Servings: 8

Ingredients:

- 8 ounces tempeh, cut into ½ -inch pieces
- 1 (2-ounce) jar chopped pimientos, drained
- ¼ cup nutritional yeast
- ¼ cup vegan mayonnaise, homemade or store-bought
- 2 tablespoons soy sauce
- ¾ cup chopped pecans

Directions:

1. Cook the tempeh within 30 minutes in a medium saucepan of simmering water. Set aside to cool. In a food processor, combine the cooled tempeh, pimientos, nutritional yeast, mayo, and soy sauce. Process until smooth.
2. Transfer the tempeh mixture to a bowl and refrigerate until firm and chilled for at least 2 hours or overnight.
3. Toast the pecans in a dry skillet over medium heat until lightly toasted. Set aside to cool.

4. Shape the tempeh batter into a ball, then roll it in the pecans, pressing the nuts slightly into the tempeh mixture so they stick. Refrigerate within 1 hour before serving.

Nutrition: Calories: 170 Carbs: 6g Fat: 14g Protein: 5g

44. Peppers and Hummus

Preparation time: 15 minutes

Cooking time: 0 minutes

Servings: 4

Ingredients:

- one 15-ounce can chickpeas, drained and rinsed
- juice of 1 lemon, or 1 tablespoon prepared lemon juice
- ¼ cup tahini
- 3 tablespoons extra-virgin olive oil
- ½ teaspoon ground cumin
- 1 tablespoon water
- ¼ teaspoon paprika
- 1 red bell pepper, sliced
- 1 green bell pepper, sliced
- 1 orange bell pepper, sliced

Directions:

1. Combine chickpeas, lemon juice, tahini, 2 tablespoons of the olive oil, the cumin, and water in a food processor.
2. Process on high speed until blended for about 30 seconds. Scoop the hummus into a bowl and drizzle with the remaining tablespoon of olive oil.

3. Sprinkle with paprika and serve with sliced bell peppers.

Nutrition: Calories: 170 Carbs: 13g Fat: 12g Protein: 4g

SMOOTHIES AND JUICES

45. <u>Sweet and Sour Juice</u>

Preparation time: 5 minutes

Cooking time: 0 minute

Servings: 2

Ingredients:

- 2 medium apples, cored, peeled, chopped
- 2 large cucumbers, peeled
- 4 cups chopped grapefruit
- 1 cup mint

Directions:

1. Process all the ingredients in the order in a juicer or blender and then strain it into two glasses.
2. Serve straight away.

Nutrition: Calories: 90 Cal Fat: 0 g Carbs: 23 g Protein: 0 g Fiber: 9 g

46. Green Lemonade

Preparation time: 5 minutes

Cooking time: 0 minute

Servings: 2

Ingredients:

- 10 large stalks of celery, chopped
- 2 medium green apples, cored, peeled, chopped
- 2 medium cucumbers, peeled, chopped
- 2 inches' piece of ginger
- 10 stalks of kale, chopped
- 2 cups parsley

Directions:

1. Process all the ingredients in the order in a juicer or blender and then strain it into two glasses.
2. Serve straight away.

Nutrition: Calories: 102.3 Cal Fat: 1.1 g Carbs: 26.2 g Protein: 4.7 g Fiber: 8.5 g

DESSERT

47. <u>Blueberry Hand Pies</u>

Preparation time: 15 minutes

Cooking time: 20 minutes

Servings: 6-8

Ingredients:

- 3 cups all-purpose flour, + extra for dusting work surface
- ½ teaspoon salt
- ¼ cup, plus 2 tablespoons granulated sugar, divided
- 1 cup vegan butter
- ½ cup cold water
- 1 cup fresh blueberries
- 2 teaspoons lemon zest
- 2 teaspoons lemon juice
- ¼ teaspoon ground cinnamon
- 1 teaspoon cornstarch
- ¼ cup unsweetened soy milk
- Coarse sugar, for sprinkling

Directions:

1. Warm your oven to 375°F. Prepare a large baking sheet lined using parchment paper. Set aside.

2. In a large bowl, combine the flour, salt, 2 tablespoons of granulated sugar, and vegan butter. Using a pastry cutter or two knives moving in a crisscross pattern, cut the butter into the other ingredients until the butter is the size of small peas.

3. Put the cold water then knead to form a dough. Tear the dough in half and wrap the halves separately in plastic wrap. Refrigerate for 15 minutes.

4. Make the blueberry filling. In a medium bowl, combine the blueberries, lemon zest, lemon juice, cinnamon, cornstarch, and the remaining ¼ cup of sugar.

5. Remove one half of the dough. On a floured surface, roll out the dough to ¼- to ½-inch thickness. Turn a 5-inch bowl upside down, and, using it as a guide, cut the dough into circles to make mini pie crusts.

6. Reroll scrap dough to cut out more circles. Repeat with the second half of the dough. You should end up with 10 to 12 circles. Place the circles on the prepared sheet pan.

7. Spoon 1½ tablespoons of blueberry filling onto each circle, leaving a ¼-inch border. Fold the circles in half to cover the filling, forming a half-moon shape. Press the edges of your dough to seal the pies using a fork.

8. When all the pies are assembled, use a paring knife to score the pies by cutting three lines through the top crusts.

9. Brush each pie with soy milk and sprinkle with coarse sugar. Bake for 20 minutes or until the filling is bubbly and the tops are golden. Let cool before serving.

Nutrition: Calories: 416Fat: 23 gCarbs: 46 gProtein: 6 g

48. <u>Date Squares</u>

Preparation time: 15 minutes

Cooking time: 25 minutes

Servings: 12

Ingredients:

- Cooking spray, for greasing
- 1½ cups rolled oats
- 1½ cups all-purpose flour
- ¾ cup, + 1/3 cup brown sugar, divided
- ½ teaspoon ground cinnamon
- ¼ teaspoon ground nutmeg
- 1 teaspoon baking soda
- ¼ teaspoon salt
- ¾ cup vegan butter
- 18 pitted dates
- 1 teaspoon lemon zest
- 1 teaspoon lemon juice
- 1 cup water

Directions:

1. Preheat the oven to 350°F. Oiled or spray a 9-inch square baking dish. Set aside.
2. Make the base and topping mixture. In a large bowl, combine the rolled oats, flour, ¾ cup of brown sugar, cinnamon, nutmeg, baking soda, and salt.
3. Add the butter and, using a pastry cutter or two knives working in a crisscross motion, cut the butter into the mixture to form a crumbly dough. Press half of your dough into the prepared baking dish and set the remaining half aside.
4. For the date filling, place a small saucepan over medium heat. Add the dates, the remaining 1/3 cup of sugar, the lemon zest, lemon juice, and water. Boil and cook within 7 to 10 minutes, until thickened.
5. When cooked, pour the date mixture over the dough base in the baking dish and top with the remaining crumb dough.
6. Gently press down and spread evenly to cover all the filling. Bake for 25 minutes until lightly golden on top. Cool before serving. Store in an airtight container.

Nutrition: Calories: 443Fat: 12 g Carbs: 81 g Protein: 5 g

49. <u>**Watermelon Lollies**</u>

Preparation Time: 15 minutes

Cooking Time: 0 minutes

Servings: 5

Ingredients:

- ½ cup watermelon, cubed
- 2 tablespoons lemon juice, freshly squeezed
- ½ cup water
- 1 tablespoon stevia

Directions:

1. In a food processor, put cubed watermelon. Process until smooth. Divide an equal amount of the mixture into an ice pop container.
2. Place inside the freezer for 1 hour.
3. Meanwhile, in a small bowl, put together lemon juice, water, and stevia.
4. Mix well. Pour over frozen watermelon lollies.
5. Add in pop sticks. Freeze for another hour.

6. Pry out watermelon lollies.
7. Serve.

Nutrition: Calories: 90 Carbs: 19g Fat: 1g Protein: 1g

50. <u>**Orange Blueberry Blast**</u>

Preparation Time: 30 minutes

Cooking Time: 0 minute

Servings: 1

Ingredients:

- 1 cup almond milk
- 1 scoop plant-based protein powder
- 1 cup blueberries
- 1 orange, peeled
- 1 teaspoon nutmeg
- 1 tablespoon shredded coconut

Directions:

1. Add all ingredients to a blender. Hit the pulse button and blend till it is smooth. Chill well to serve.

Nutrition Calories: 155 Carbs: 12g Fat: 21g Protein: 1g